GOSSIPING WITH MY EMOTIONS

SONAL MAHARANA

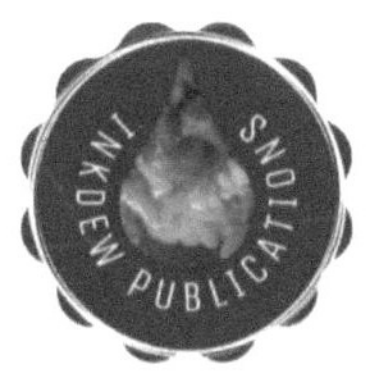

GOSSIPING WITH MY EMOTIONS

DIVING DEEP INTO THE HEART

SONAL MAHARANA

First Published by
INKDEW PRIVATE LIMITED

Title of the book : Gossiping with my emotions
Sonal Maharana
Copyright ©Sonal Maharana, 2021
ISBN 9788195331338

Cover design : **Gaurav Maharana**
Line arts credit www.pixabay.com

Printed in India
PRICE Rs 150.00 INDIA, $15 ABROAD

INKDEW PRIVATE LIMITED
Pujariguda, Chandahandi
Nabarangpur, Odisha - 764077

WE ARE AVAILABLE ON
https://www.inkdew.com
Email : info@inkdew.com
mob: +91 6371119094

Preface

To all those who find it difficult to understand their emotions...

I know emotions are to be felt, not understood. But feeling weird emotions without understanding them is like moving on a speeding car without brakes. You can go on feeling the pain or feeling bizarre almost lifelong without recognizing which emotion you're going through and when. When you know your emotions, it's easy to deal with them, especially when they play havoc in your mind.

In this book, all the emotions are personified. A dialogue with them is initiated. Then they are accused or appreciated for their roles. The readers are requested to create an imaginary picture of each of their emotions standing right in front of them. Please stop after each stanza. Let it sink in your mind completely before heading to the next one.

Then you can bombard your idiosyncratic questions on their particular emotions. The poetry may end in pages but the dialogues must not end till there's a winner between the reader and the particular emotion of his or her. Even if there's no winner, a resolution for peace of mind must be the agenda. In addition to this, there are these 10 rare emotions that we all go through sometimes or the other.

But, we hardly realize what this feeling is actually. For example, 'Sonder' is a rare emotion where there is a realization that everyone has a story. 'Monachopsis' is that weird feeling that you're out of place. These poetic pages are not just pages. They are some or the other corners of my heart where melodic beats whisper different auras into my ears. And then the whole body is drenched in them.

This work is inspired by the cluttered mind that I used to experience at one point in my life. So many emotions were taking a roller-coaster ride through the wires (neurons) of the brain. One moment felt euphoric, the other was so gloomy. So many questions, few were the answers.

Then, the roller-coaster had to take a break when this mind started practising some spiritual activities (particularly Rajyog meditation taught by the Brahmakumaris spiritual university). For a change, a clear canvas with clear images of those mysterious emotions was painted. And a beautiful picture called 'Life' was made.

This picture was then destined to take the shape of poetry.

And thus, 'Gossiping with my emotions' was born.

Acknowledgement

The first book of my life. A dream came true. Thank you Life, thank you Destiny. Thank you to all the faces that led me through these emotions that are described in the book.

The first share of thanks in every aspect of life is, was and always will be for The Almighty God (whom I lovingly call Shivbaba). 'Thank you Shivbaba, thanks a lot.'

Then, the following people deserve an equal share of thanks for making 'Gossiping with my Emotions' possible for me.

Thank you to my parents Sarpeswar Maharana and Subasini Maharana for being wonderful and encouraging parents. Thanks, Mummy, Papa for never saying 'You're a girl, you can't do it. But, you always said 'You're a girl, you can definitely do it.'.

Special thanks to my husband Sitendu Maharana for always being the pillar of my life and tolerating me when I tunnelled myself to that solitude space. I would also like to thank him here for being my biggest critic suggesting some edits with great accuracy.
Special thanks to my brother Gaurav Maharana who helped me in every possible way with his invaluable suggestions. The cover page and the designs included in this book showcase your immense brilliance in whatever you take up.

Special thanks to the angel of my life, my daughter Shreeanshi Maharana (Nimi) whose smiles, cries, tantrums all inspired me to experience several emotions.

Special thanks to Manoj Sir for being able to unwrap the poet in me and pushing me consistently to deliver my best.

Special thanks to all my family members for inspiring me to experience all those weird emotions through their ones.

Special thanks to my childhood friends Nivya Velayudhan, Hetal Sheth and Sanghmitra Shah for being my friend when I was naive about the word 'friend'.

Special thanks to my dear friends (Gautambhai, Nidhi, Jyotibhai, Asmita, Dillipbhai, Rashmita, Pankajbhai, Neha, Devbhai, Rajani) for their consistent encouraging words. Truly, we'll always be 'Friends forever'.
Special thanks to Ruchi and Koustuvbhai for their affirmative vibrancy. Special thanks to Arpita Mishra, a chance meeting with whom in train led to a life-long friendship.

Lastly, a ton of thanks to all the subscribers of my YouTube channel 'Spiritual Dose 4U' for their faith in this atypical channel of mine.

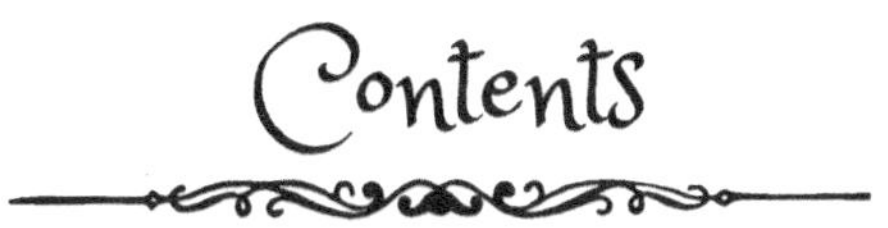 Contents

Part I : General Emotions

Part II : Rare Emotions

Part III : Self-Test for Emotional Quotient

You may have experienced those.
But you may not know.
You may have wondered about their strange flow.
But you may not know.
Let's know them now.
Let's start the emotional journey now.
Let's break free and dive deep into the heart.

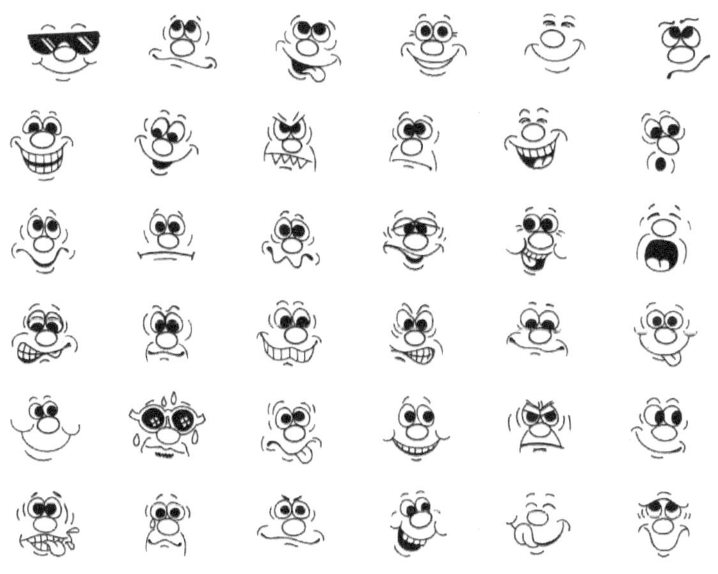

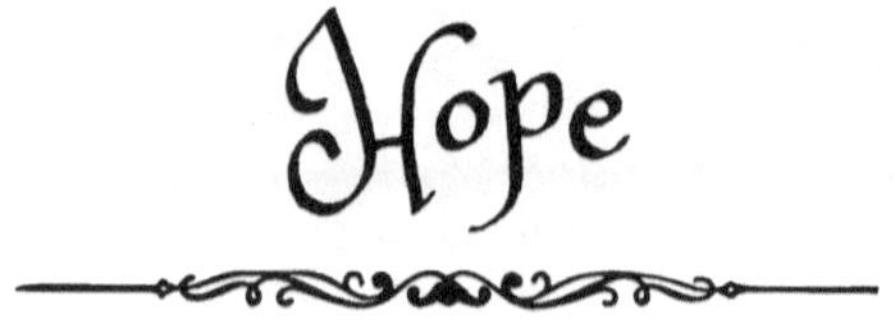

Hope

A drowning man grasps at a straw. You're the straw.
A sinking sweetheart swiftly rises. You're the elevator.
A vanishing scenery shows up in a flash. You're the
spotlight beam.

Only one utterance for you, That's 'Thank you.'
Thank you, You're there.
For every repair.
When it's tough to bear.
To melt down all the despair.
And hold hands for a prayer.
Even when life is unfair.
You grant that dare.
To wipe out the last tear,
And the face glows again with that glare!

They call me sightless when I'm with You. But I love this
darkness!
When it's the gateway to the approaching source of
luminousness.

They call me doltish to trust the impossible.
I say You're the one responsible.

They call me outlandish to take the path less traveled
I say, it's for a universal bloom that ought to be
channeled!

This is my endeavour.
You stay with me forever.
You stay with me forever.

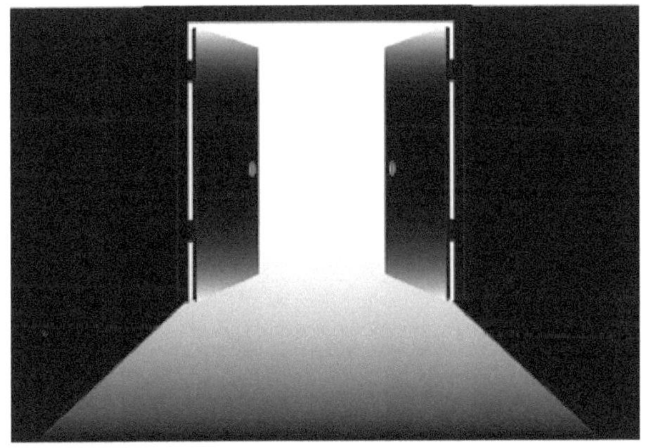

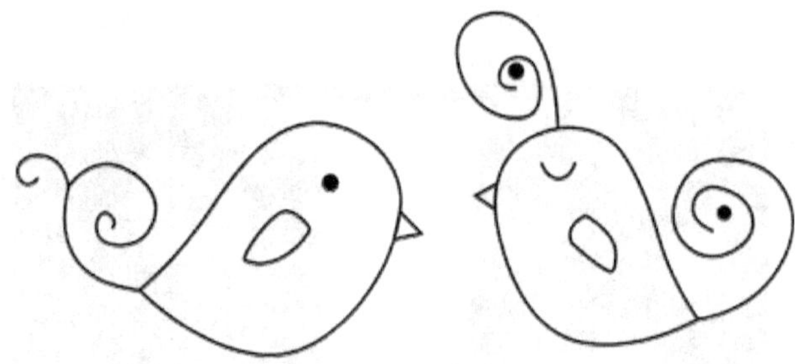

Gossiping with my emotions

4

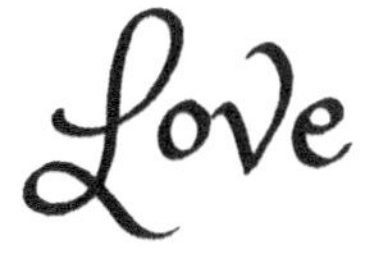

Love

Four-letter word and an ocean of Euphoria!
Four-letter word and an ocean of Ecstasy!
Four-letter word and an ocean of tears!

You drenched my heart, You drenched my soul.
You're also an ocean of power, An ocean of might
That can move mountains, perform miracles,
resolve any fight!

Your sweet pain diffuses through me as
a mystical breeze.
Oh, I'm even more vulnerable!
You add life to those flesh and bones
Making every moment so memorable!

You offer boundless acceptance
That every soul is bound to surrender,
What a Wonder!
A matter to Ponder!
You're the pillar of life, You're at the root.
Because there's absolutely no substitute.

I plead with you today.
Please stay at every corner of my heart.
Stay there till the end of Time!
As an eternal rhyme!
As an eternal rhyme!

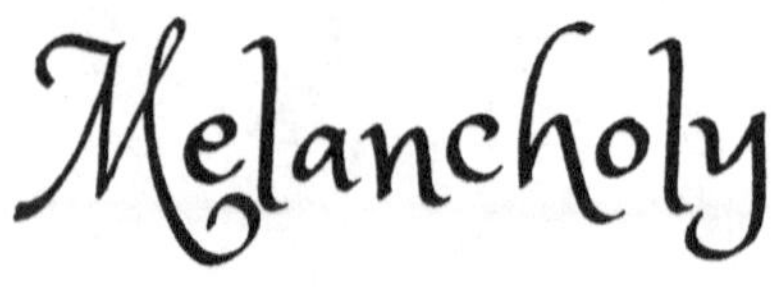

Oh! This mystical ultra poignancy!
Did I just ignore such flamboyancy?

I feel addicted to You my melancholy.
As if I'm safe from the worldly folly!

Why am I at ease with Your dark site?
Maybe to escape the brutal truth engulfed in the glow of
light!
I cannot change the world, I cannot change people, I
cannot change myself; some hassles are just born to
stay
As if You are the only way!
Sporadically, I conspire to break free from Your taut
clutch.
But instantly, Your gloomy paw gives me a touch!

Your dark hues are so ruthless
How to endure? I feel clueless!
They taunt me, lock me up in Your castle!
Where I ought to be aloof from the worldly hassle.
Where I sit with you and only You.
Aah, How lucid is this bird's eye view!
Tons of aspirations to pursue.
You accidentally ignited the fire.
As if the higher self waited to conspire!

Here, I must also confess my gratitude.
For granting me that solitude!
That metamorphosed my attitude!
To look upon at such altitude
To look upon at such altitude!

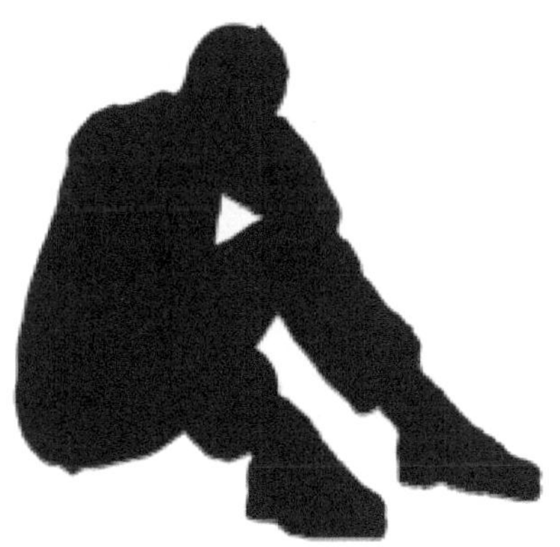

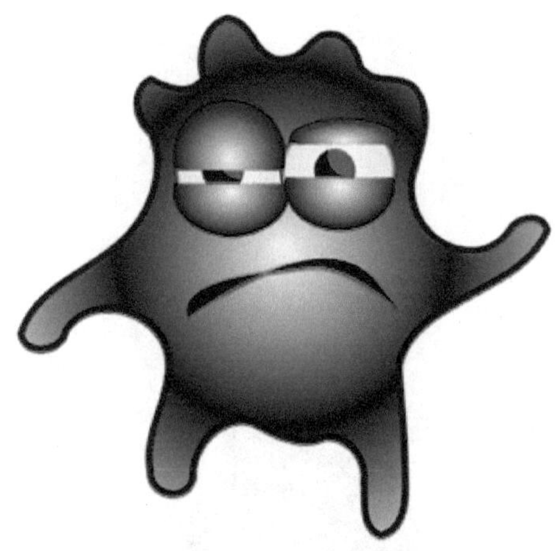

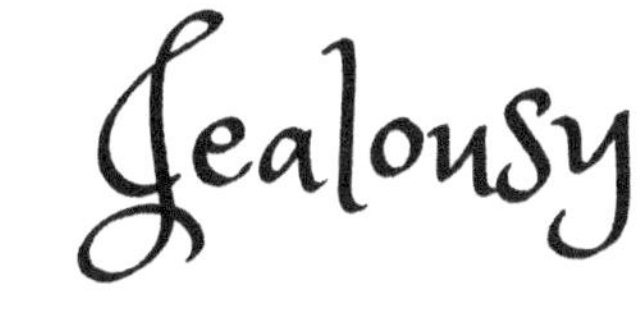

Jealousy

It's blazing, it's flickering, it's smouldering!
As if all the ardour is mouldering!

Aqua gush is an exigency!
I fear there's no insurgency!
As if the healing drizzles are the only fervency!
The drizzles of love, the drizzles of reassurance, the
drizzles of faith.
That my fella belongs to me and will be forever!
Then, all of me is presented, ready for a love swathe!

Why is it so? That every so often I'm so powerless?
You taunt me; you burn me to ashes in Your hellfire.
And I'm so powerless to backfire!

You fabricate a criminal out of me! That babbles scads
of this tosh,
Crikey! 'Oh, is it me who just thought of this hogwash?'

Will you please vent my heart? You're such a boggart!
It's time to unleash those stinging emotions like the
flowing gust,
As mine will be mine only if I shrug off the old rust.
As mine will be mine only if I shrug off the old rust.

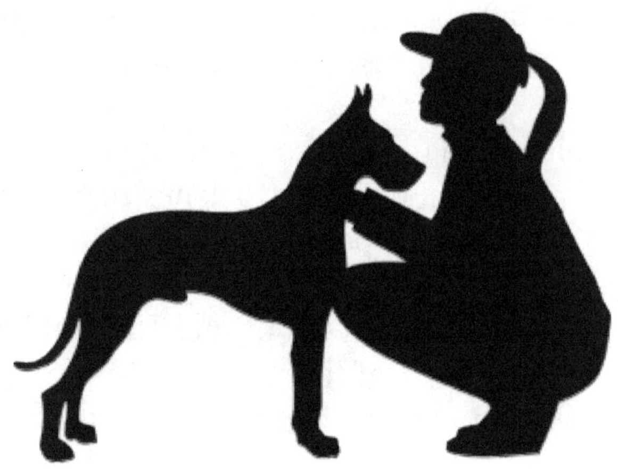

Trust

They say 'I would fall.' You assure me I won't.
I hope they believe. They don't.
Why do I believe? I know not either!

You dwell in my postulations. Are You a shadow?
The positive energies are on the flow.
All the gloom vanishes. You inject power.
There are qualms but You stand erect akin to a tower.

How enigmatic!
You're the upshot of spunk, so charismatic!
But I'm also timid. Betrayal is unbearable.
I'm skeptical. Is it repairable?
The grooves of the wounds are impressions of rock.
They go deeper and deeper after every shock!

The conscience yells at me.
'You sightless zealot! Why did you trust?'
'Now the underlying sketch is revealed, blowing up the crust!'

Alas, this heart still yearns for Your warmth.
Where is Your abode? The plethora of love!
No question of betrayal. No question of depletion.
No question of this and that era.
I suddenly stumble upon this eccentric notion.
That it lies only in the Highest Supreme.
It lies only in the Highest Supreme.

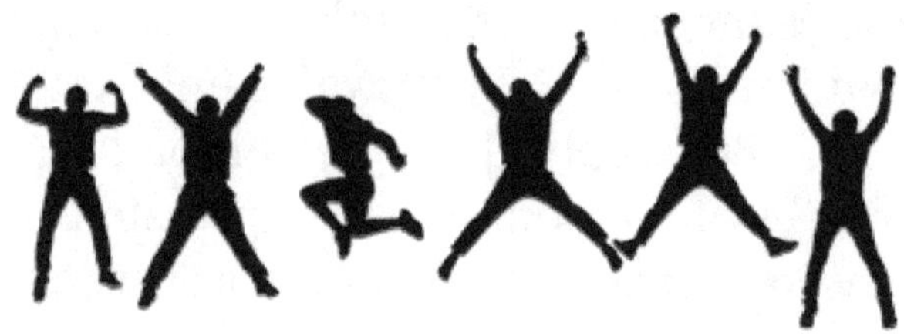

Excitement

A heart tired of all the denials refuses to desire.
Then, You spell essence to it like a medicinal vial.

The heart tries to rebel
It tries to deride, satirize
'It won't work, it'll eventually crash'
The reminiscences play in a flash.

But soon the reel transforms and I set foot in a
dreamland
The chambers of my heart begin to expand
Truly, imagination can never be planned.

Oh, what a thrill!
I'm diving into that ocean of passion
Cold shivers, butterflies around, zing are all in action.
I'm drenched with Your fierce kiss!
Hallelujah, What a bliss!

In the blink of an eye, I reject those refusals.
Since it's time for an arousal.
Triumph or a fiasco!
It's definitely time for an arousal.
It's definitely time for an arousal.

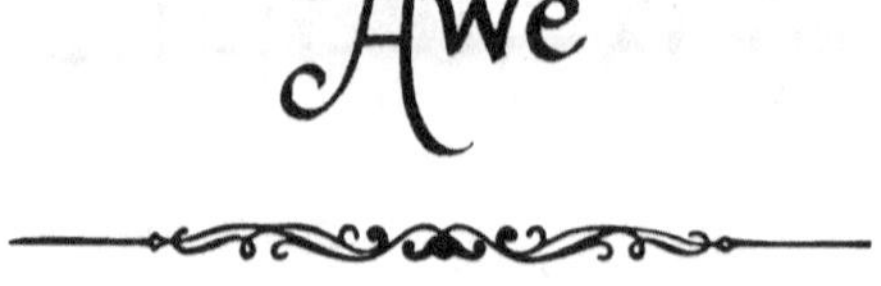

Awe

Awe! That splendid architecture.
Awe! Such a grand party.
Awe! What a breathtaking natural backdrop.
Awe! My charming beloved.

My inner core gets thrilled,
Oh, it gets chilled!
As if the euphoria is being drilled!
Every encounter with You,
Leave me with a hue!
Such intoxication!
What a sensation!
Often, it pokes me,
Like the sting of a bee!

The longing to explore more
Boundless is how much I adore.
A curious phobia encapsulates me when You're around,
Still, this heart says 'Be there, get drowned'!

It's all His Creations.
Vast is the realm of this ocean
That often is a potion!
The extravaganza of Nature perfectly synchronized
together

It Impels me to ponder its Father.
Who is behind the Creation of this Splendor?
Vast is His Creation, Vast is His Imagination, He is such
a Wonder!

His Creation is spread far and wide,
ubiquitous wherever goes my eyeball;
Zilch of a pitfall!
You are truly synonymous with Him Is my Whim!

Truly, You're there in all.
The mesmerizing hills.
The adventurous thrills.
The creations of the maven,
The imaginations of heaven!
Such boundless brilliance!
A wish for everlasting adherence
A wish for everlasting adherence!

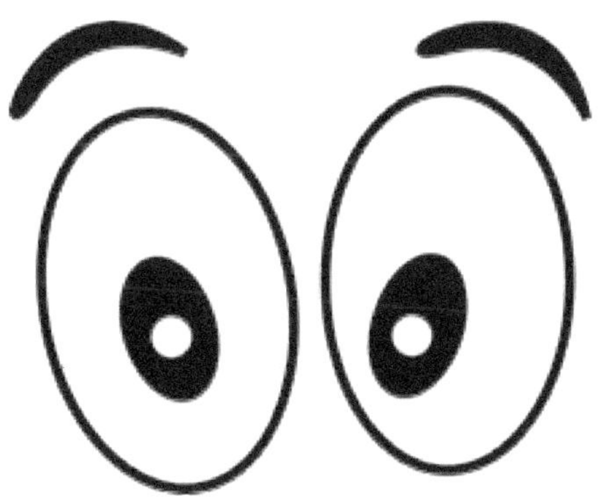

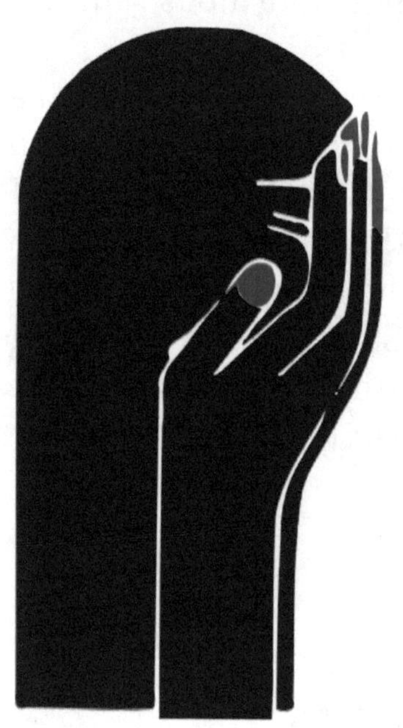

Gossiping with my emotions

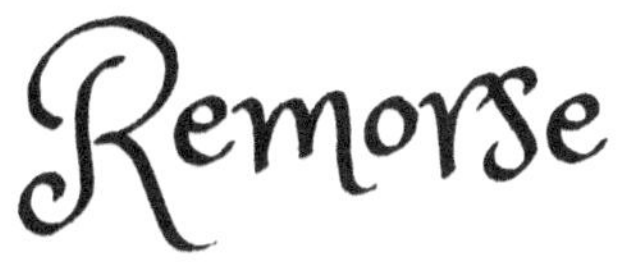

Remorse

As the deep perforating pain pinches me every
moment,
I pledge to revoke this postponement.
Postponement for a self-gazing at the mirror.
Postponement for an inner brooding.
No more of this eluding.
Eluding the past. Eluding the present.

But a glare into my eyes and the moral code fires me
up!
It accuses me of laxity,
It accuses me of scorn.
How brash of it to direct, 'Now You can mourn'!

I vindicated my innocence.
'The devil within was the culprit. That cunning
chameleon intoxicated me with his charm.'
'I was lured, being puerile about the harm!'
My plea for pardon was disapproved.
A court of the inner angel well-grooved.

Hence, I'm penalized for each instance.
And You're at work again.
In a pursuit, embellishment is Your campaign.
An embellishment of broken hearts.
Abolition of melancholy.
That sketches the alchemy of glum to jolly!
That sketches the alchemy of glum to jolly!

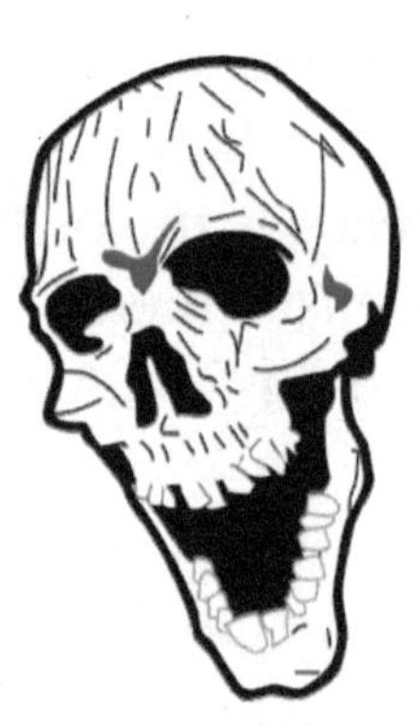

Gossiping with my emotions

18

Contempt

I'm better. I'm better any day. What a flair!
Oh, I must be gliding in the air!

Very well, they can't even touch me!
No parallel players, I love this glee!

Yes, I'm worthy of all, it's absolutely fair.
But, are they truly worthless? Do they deserve such despair?
Sure, You profess my golden heart.
But, do the silver ones ought to be torn apart?

I confess you quench me into an intoxication.
Exuberance! Exhilaration!
But, why this differentiation?
When it only confers an isolation!
Thereon, a sequel of resentment and repentance.
That's when there's a descendance!
That's when there's a descendance!

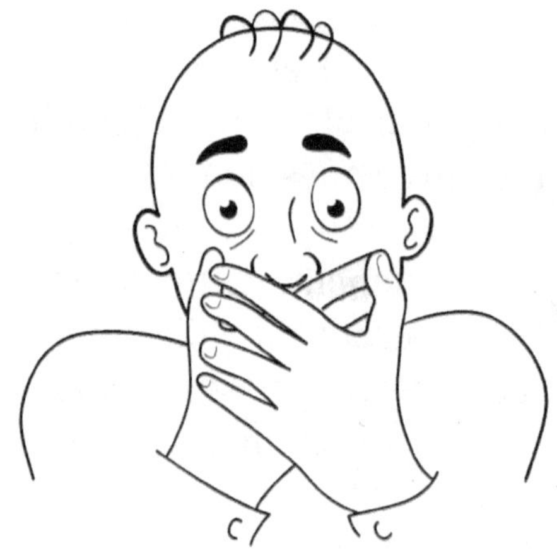

Gossiping with my emotions

20

Embarrassment

'Please don't put me in the dock for litigation,' I sighed.
You still didn't bother to subside.
Each minute of the lawsuit lasted for years.
The eyes were moist but couldn't drain out the tears.

Recurrence of such agonizing fortuity,
That sluggishly drags me to fatuity!
Then the dismay silently turns into despair,
And there it kicks down all the flair!

How cruel are You to penalize me with diffidence?
It's my innocence and Your militance!
Will you stop my sufferance?
As I doubt my resilience!

But today I know how to trounce,
For transparency is my armament, Truth is my armour.
Why shall I let You in?
When I perceive I'll win within
When I perceive I'll win within.

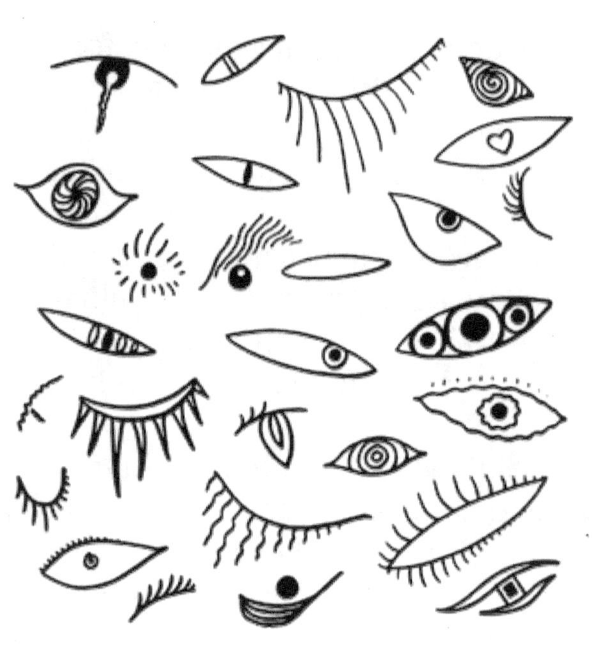

Gossiping with my emotions

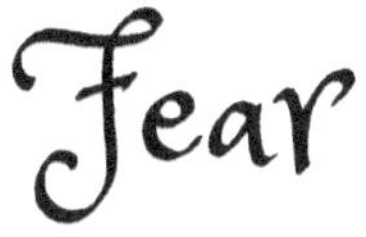

Fear

Oh, I may be vanquished!
This heart and soul will be anguished!
You haunt me on those restless nights.
Who can bear such woeful sights?
'Oh, my honey, why did you vamoose?
Now, do I have anything at all to lose?'

It's Your arrival and suddenly I'm a dud, a pauper.
Who loses all odds and ends? What a yauper!
Already impoverished in the mind's shade.
Waiting to jump out in a flash with that noted saccade.

I'm not me with You.
It's only You.
As You gulp my persona,
And transmute me to the bitterest Cinchona!

Humbly, I request You today.
Please, let me be unfettered.
Let me just shed off You like a rag.
Awaiting zealously to brag!

Yes, I'm well with the separation.
For losing You is gaining me
For losing You is gaining me.

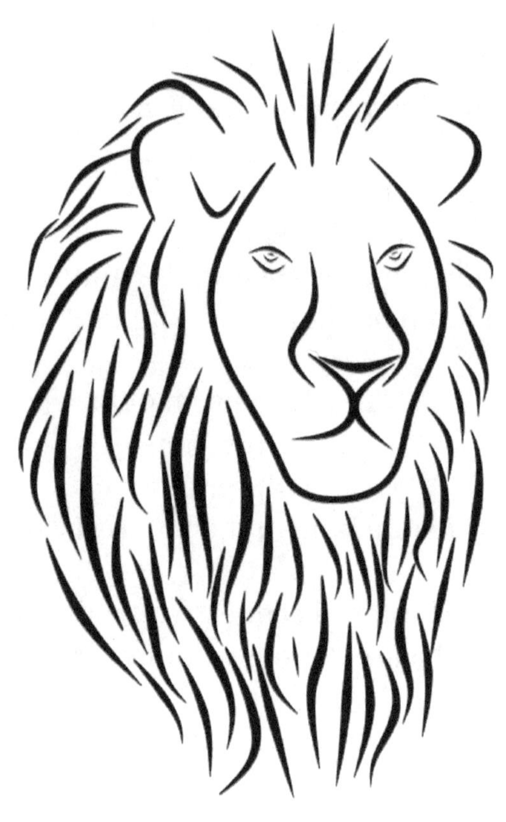

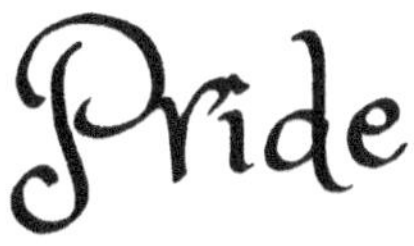

Your emergence was in a domain so tranquil.
When I was a callow juvenile to sense my will.

A Master of Camouflage, You had many faces.
How astute of You to fill those void spaces!

The creeping, descending confidence inclined to a
surge.
And that was You who yearned to emerge.
Under-confidence transmuted into overconfidence!
Eventually, You were under prominence.

Such a con, aren't You? Who loves to be under the veil.
Although a hooligan, You're the shield of the frail!

Oh, You made me so imperceptive
who could only see the 'I',
That often lumbered me to such an awful sigh!

Designated as amour propre, dignity or You;
Are You my Saviour or Satan?
Are You my Saviour or Satan?

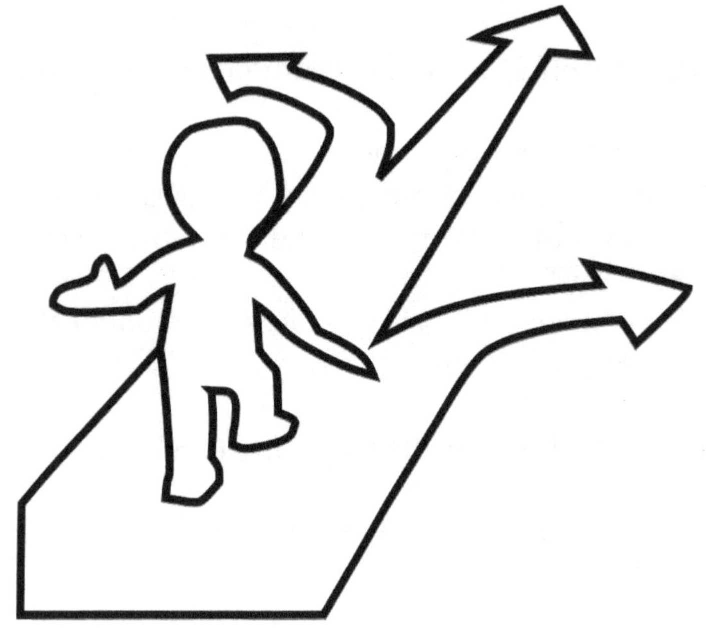

Confusion

Those cyclonic swirls, a giant whirlwind in the head.
This or that?
What a combat!

The giants striving to crush each other,
It's a confrontation. Brawl, they smother!
Oh my, dearie me! Does anyone even bother?

You compel me to set off as a beggar!
Beggar of prospects, beggar of assuagements, beggar of
an affirmation.
For all my standpoints are in cremation!

Gosh, it's pathetic!
A confused bullhead who can easily be fed
With all the tittle-tattles, all that is so dead!
A beggar to a patsy, how miserable!
Truly, inexplicable. How vulnerable!

Free-willed, unbiased, lucid.
Some attributes I awfully aspire to.
Some attributes I awfully aspire to.

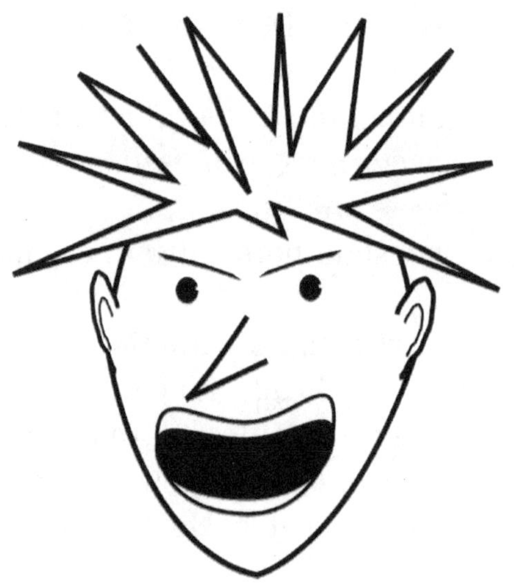

Frustration

A freakish wish often falls into this void
Let me just fly off!
Fly off to the sky, Fly off to the moon,
Fly off to the infinite,
Fly off to the mysterious!

Fly off ceaselessly.
What an Odyssey! Such a liberation!

Why endure?
When it's all in vain!
Why to cajole?
When there's an internal refrain!

It's all over in a moment,
Exorbitant emotional quotient!
All these years were a waste,
I wish they could be erased!

Although You're least adorable to embrace,
I hardly possess anything to replace!
Oh, the familiar disgrace!
It's the heart's fireplace!
It's the heart's fireplace!

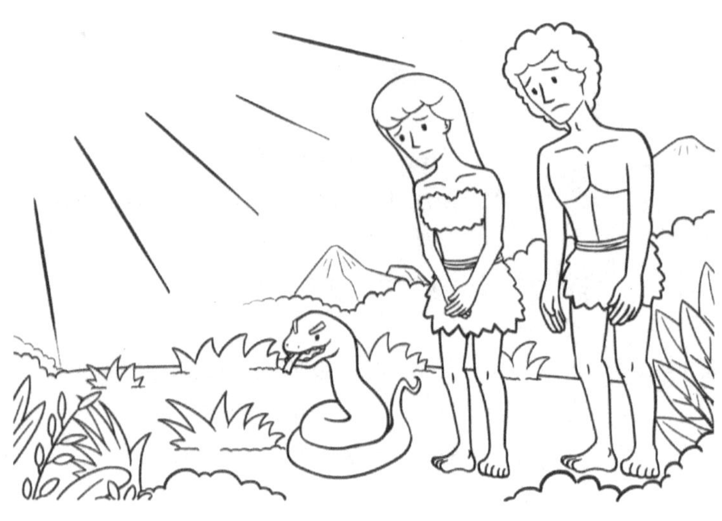

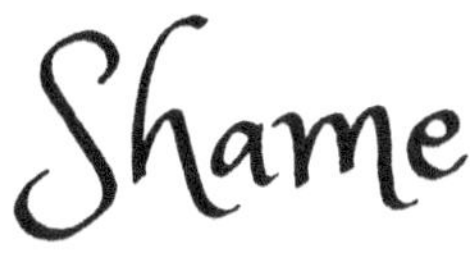

Shame

Embarrassment! Remorse!
Oh, You must be over the moon!
Once more You've poached me, I feel like a loon!

The consistent blunders!
The inexhaustible stockpile of gaffes!
The resultant incessant self-monologue!
When will this intellect learn from its awful catalogue?

How can I dodge You?
As the dreadful pinching pain haunts,
You are always there to flaunt!

Perplexed at the verdicts of this feeble mind,
How imprudent? Is it blind!
Cluttered intentions, freaky actions
Were those any sort of conspiration?
And You can set Your foot in
With a huge grin
Momentarily, this heart exclaims,
'jilt into the bin, jilt into the bin!'

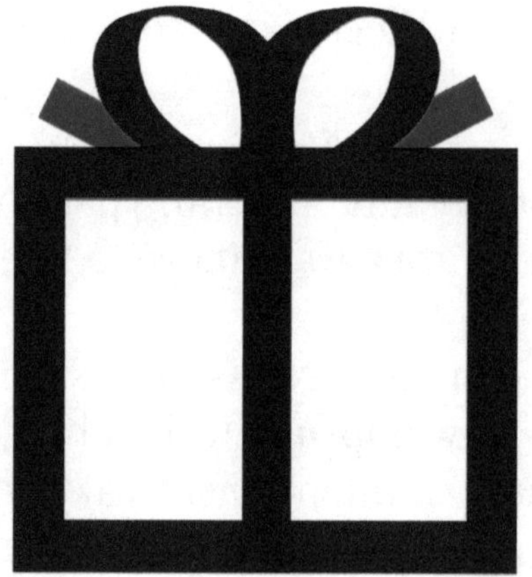

Surprise

Astonished, flabbergasted, stunned!
You're such a sorcerer!
One moment and there's this gigantic upturn.
The eyes are wide-open,
The body gets those chills running down the spine!
And You're still revealing Yourself so slothfully!

As if a fantasy awakens.
Oh! The identical sight.
A mystifying delight!

Is it a hallucination?
Or Your incredible power of fascination?

But, why do You at times transmute to a black tint?
What despair!
A pally sorcerer to a tyrant! Is it fair?

Thoughts coming alive as a reality!
At times, it's predestination,
At times, it's my contemplation,
The architect of such a variation!
Sometimes, gratification
Sometimes, exasperation!

Prithee, Let me be in that deep stillness.
And just be a silent witness.
And just be a silent witness.

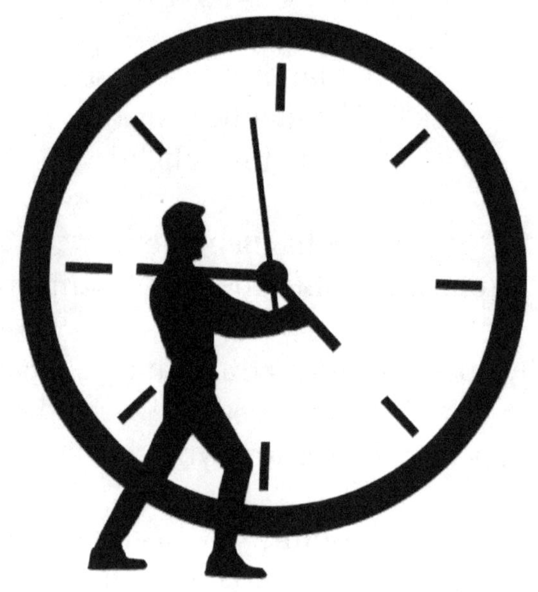

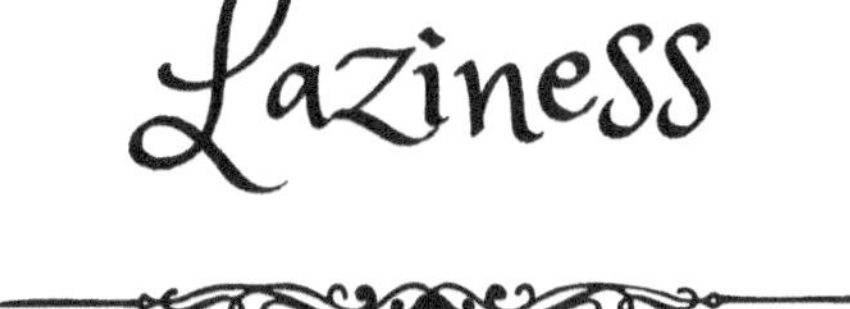

Laziness

Oh, my best buddy for a while now
Though separation is never serene,
Can You please evacuate my heart screen?

Why are You so fond of getting glued to me?
A sudden adrenaline kick,
And there's an abrupt prick
'Oh, You fool! It's time to doze'
I heard Your shrieking voice and froze!

It's so erratic to feel You amid an elation
The heart craves to solve a puzzle
But, all the zeal gets splintered like a bubble
Once You greet it with a cuddle!

For some, You're a leisure
For me, You're indolence!

Though You act innocent,
I've discovered You as a foe in disguise
Who's envious of my rise!

I crave that cryptic yearning
For a child-like zest in every tick
Please evacuate my heart flowing like a foul slick!
Please evacuate my heart flowing like a foul slick!

Self-Pity

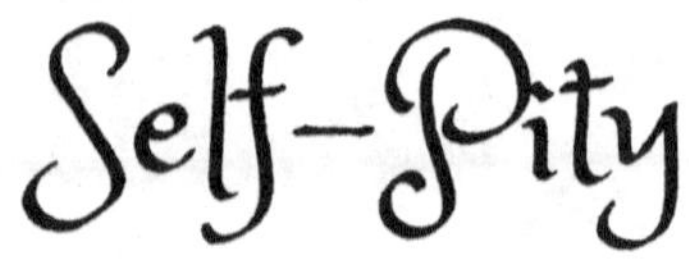

All the amenities, all the assistance, still a void?

Poor me! Oh me!
Alas, Woe to me!

A constant assistance, a constant aid
A comfort zone I refuse to annihilate,
An unenviable trait.
Desperate for an unceasing helping hand,
You invariably curb me to expand.

The past burdens of innocent delinquencies
Are up for a screenplay. Oh, such scary contingencies!
Whenever I get entangled in an ocean of emotions.
Whenever I can't rescue myself out of it.

But, all the hitches appear minuscule
At the sight of a heart-piercing scene,
A scene of a poor vulnerable woman
A scene of a child being exploited brutally
A scene of a heroic soldier's funeral

Although skeptical, I wish for the arrival of a day
When there will be
Self-pity to self-empowerment
Poor me to wow me!
Weakness to strength
A journey from darkness to light
Ceaseless aspirations, but why such hesitation!
Ceaseless aspirations, but why such hesitation!

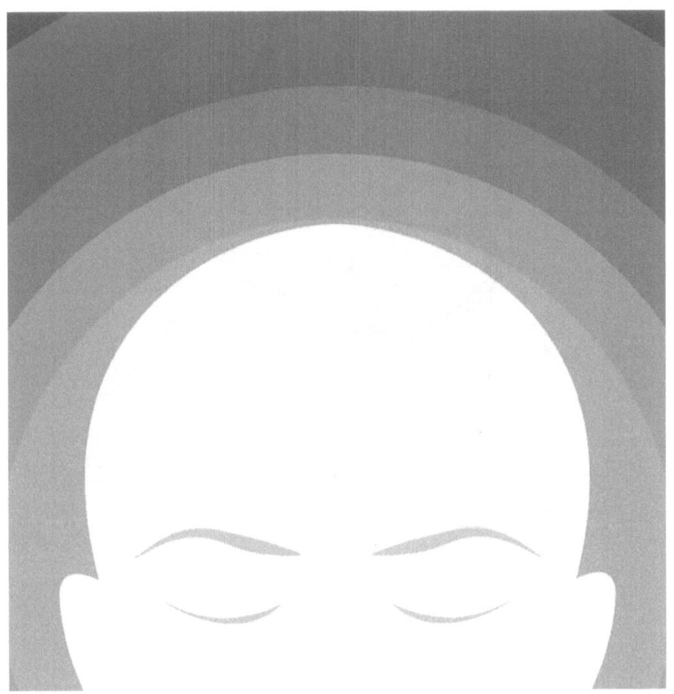

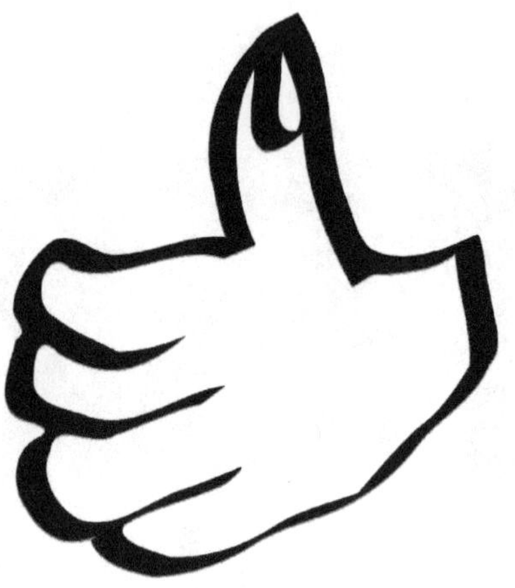

Satisfaction

You emerge in this heart in several instances.
Here are some to recall and rejoice.

An inexplicable smile on this face when it disperses a
ton of smiles.
A brimful tummy when the hands make some
brimmed.

The devil inside says 'What a loss!'
You say, 'A price for this facial gloss!'
You quickly fill my heart with your warmth.
That soon diffuses out to bestow the bliss henceforth.

They enquire, 'Why so much exertion?'
You're their answer.
They work for money. I work for You.
I'm naive about my wages. They're naive about You.

I confess I'm stupid, I'm insane!
But, such a delight, how can I explain?
You inject it into my blood with every letter on paper.
And all the qualms get evaporated like vapour.

I wish You linger here perpetually.
But off and on, You get hijacked by the devil!
Such a tug of war, then I ought to play!
Such a tug of war, then I ought to play!

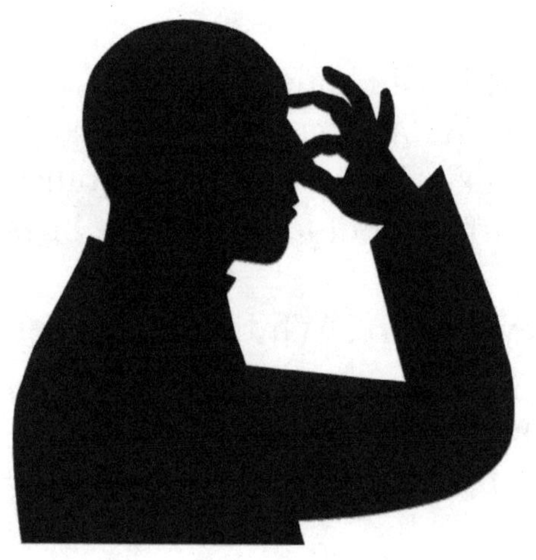

Gossiping with my emotions

Disgust

You pop up in my heart whenever it bumps into an
injustice.
You pop up in my heart at the very sight of inveracity
and bigotry
To hell with these worldly norms that only brings about
asymmetry!

Why let go, why ignore when it only strengthens the
repetition?
Surrendering before the unjust, believing a fiction, such
a contradiction!

The bandit clan feels splendid about thyself, no angst or
an intent to transform
The Dance of hypocrisy, the approach of a Hailstorm
Here's a menacing laugh, there's a deep mourning!

The Golden hearts are in grief, the stone hearts are
rejoicing
What a scene!
Felony of the wolverine!
Let me close my eyes, can't view this catastrophe
anymore
But, how to ignore, how to shut the heart door?
It's your peak now! The crest is sobbing too!
Even worse.
Being handcuffed, there's nothing I can do!
Truly, There's nothing I can do!

Inferiority Complex

I warrant myself 'I'm nothing.' 'I'm nothing apropos of
them.'
I curiously ask about it's truth?
You give your final verdict 'Yes, it is true!'
I'm shattered, I'm shocked, I'm distressed!
You ruthlessly linger on your words.
I defy.
You quell the traces of confidence in me.
I beg for your mercy.
You defy.
I mourn.
You scorn.

How can You be so still?
When I shrill!
Congratulations! That You've successfully buried a
genius!
Oh, What a conspiracy!
Why is it perpetually Your Supremacy?

You always spurn my peculiarities.
Intolerant to such disparities!
How ignorant to ignore the polarities?

But I also took a pledge today.
A pledge to uproot you out.
A pledge to extinguish your very presence.
A pledge to vanquish you.
For I realize that I play my role, they play theirs.
It's all about our unique affairs.
It's all about our unique affairs.

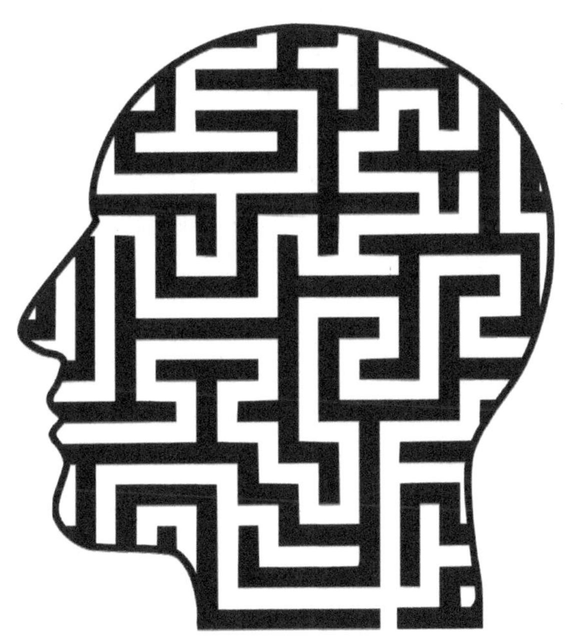

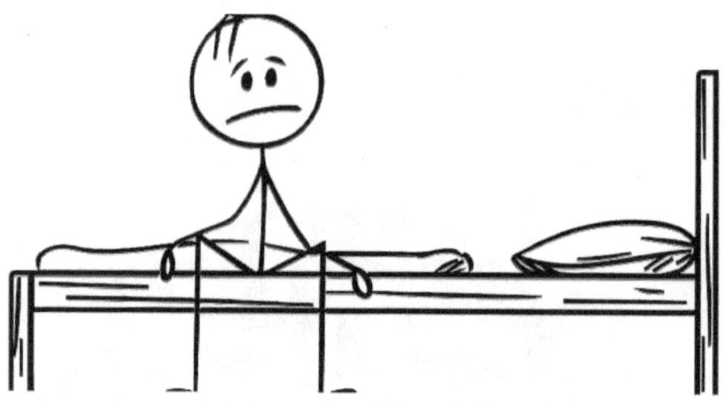

Gossiping with my emotions

Loneliness

Encompassed with zillions of faces.
All are bizarre! Wandering in alien spaces!

Isn't it weird like Your pungent taste?
As if all is a waste!

Lonely as a desert tree
Lonely as a ship in the Ocean
Apparently, stillness in motion!
Lonely with a slew of lights around!
Still so dark! An episode that never fails to astound.

They fail to enlighten the darkness of this heart!
Warmth in the eyes, palsy-walsy vibes, so many wishes
in the cart.

Lonely with a void inside!
The inaudible space where You love to hide.
Even the chatterbox within is so silent today!
Seems as if all is swept away!
Seems as if all is swept away!

Compassion

The thirsty tongue,
The awaiting arms
Moist eyes of a mother,
Paralyzed hands of a father.
The mourns of a child
The silent sigh of a wife
How iffy is life!

All piled up in my heart that it's so hefty now.
The scenes I cannot expunge
The heroic benefactor is up to take a plunge
The screams scream in my ears too
To bring back the nightly snores is what I pursue!

You make me feel their agony.
You make me suffer with them.
But, you also arouse me for a revolution.
Thus, I'm up for a resolution.

Oh! What a pain! What distress!
Distressed with such silence!
What endurance!
And here goes some babbling.
How to be the voice of those voiceless martyrs?
How to reinforce power in them?
When will they learn to fight the mayhem?

A fight is vital.
A fight with that inner feeble being.
A fight with that outer vicious world.
Waiting for the kick-off.
Waiting for the upheaval!
Waiting for the rebellion!
And also the tranquillity that'll follow.
That stuffs up all the hollow!

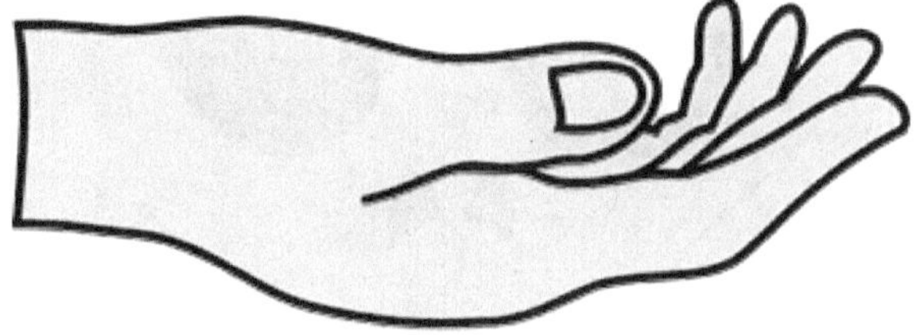

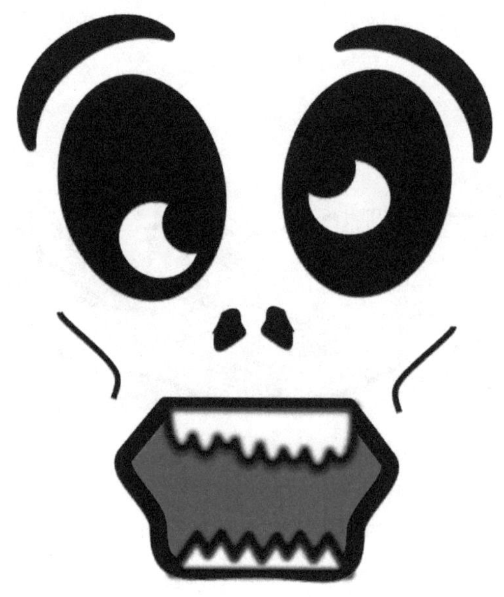

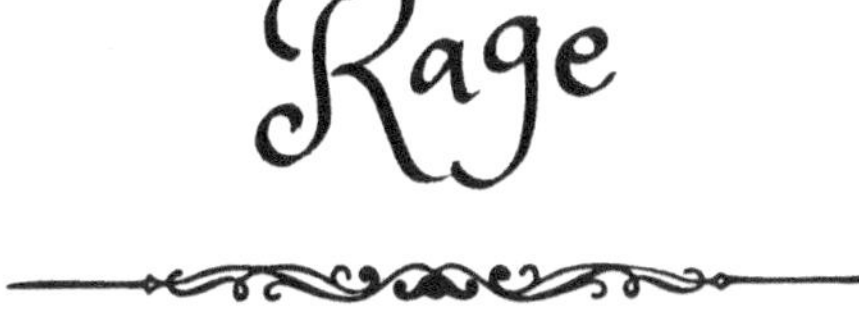

You silently step into my heart
I'm utterly naive about you.
Till this hasty rush of emotions!
That crops up as an implosion!
And then that pally jumbled up fervour of guilt!
What an inveterate conflict!
Oh, that blasé act!
Hope I can retract.

I object to the bias, I object to the bigotry, I object to the inequality.
Hope to inculcate some frivolity!

Accept, let go, forget and forgive; arduous tasks for this bolshie heart!
Wish to learn this novel art!

I often dream
Of a day of triumph
Of Indifference over Rage,
Of Calmness over Restlessness,
Of Love over Hatred
Being Upbeat, Being sanguine
May my dream be a reality, Amen!
May my dream be a reality, Amen!

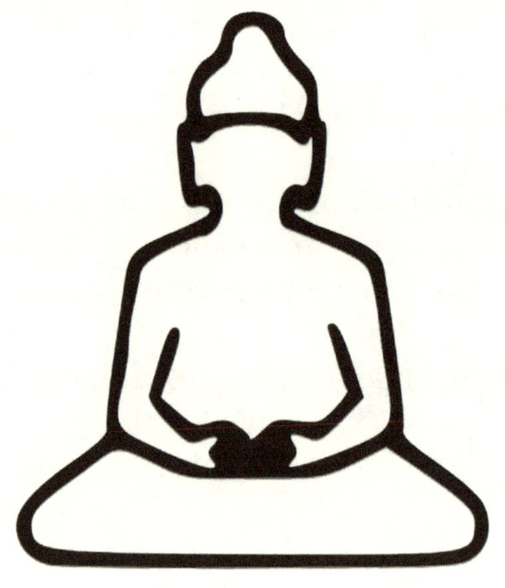

Contentment

Love those beautiful flowers
But do I yearn for them?
Love those mouth-watering delicacies.
But do I yearn for them?
Love those lavish assets
But do I yearn for them?

'Love' doesn't metamorphose to 'Want'
A voice within screams 'Why to flaunt?'
Such a weird feeling of satiety!
Why do You induce that bizarre sobriety?

There's peace within, there's happiness, it's so calm
I'm at liberty. What's the need of any qualm?

Some possess all but You.
I possess You but all.
Where do I go with that hefty haul!

Wants are eternal, ceaseless endeavours
Jumbled up in malevolent fervours!

O my Contented heart,
Why don't you allure those possessions, be an astute
being?
Your pat answer from it where You indwell,
'You can only have one, either those assets or just me!'
'You can only have one, either those assets or just me!'

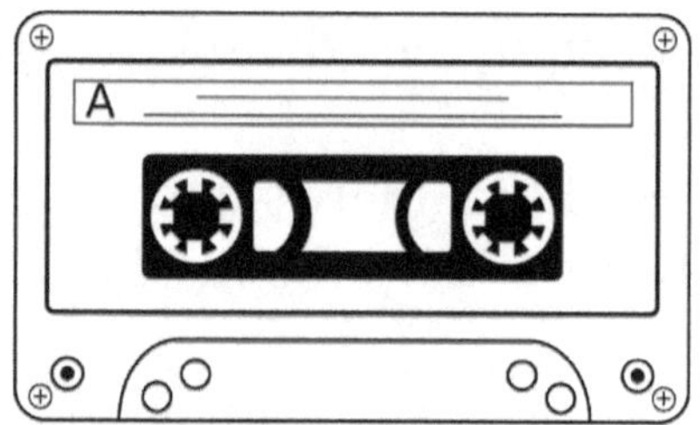
A

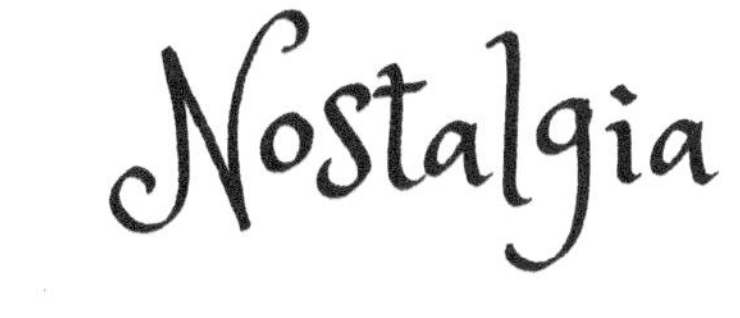

Nostalgia

'Those were the days.' 'That was the era.' 'That was life.'

'Dynamic, Vibrant, Vivacious.'

You always whisper in my ears.
As if You loathe my contemporary peers.
I can sense Your zealous intentions,
As You breeze in silently through the doors of my
attention!

Oh, a fabulous feeling!
With the heart lingering in the bygone days.
Then, this realization that it was only a phase!
The rush of grief once I resurge into the here and now!
It's only this horrible poignancy,
Could You please show some leniency?

O my beloved Nostalgia, wave me goodbye
As I shun You today!
I shun you today as You leave me yearning!
I shun you today as You leave me aghast!
I shun you today as You leave me rattled!

Though I ought to shun You from my consciousness,
What about my unconscious souvenirs?
Though I ought to tiptoe into the futurity,
You succeed to flinch me back to that propensity!
You succeed to flinch me back to that propensity!

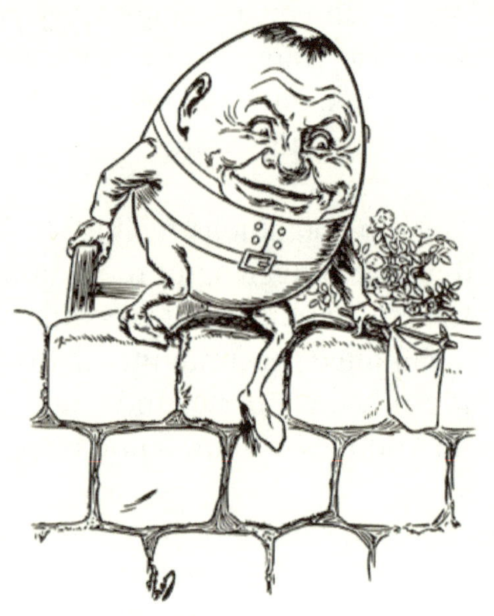

Gossiping with my emotions

Amusement

You are the colours of this canvas called Life!
How vivid! How flamboyant!
How brilliant! How dramatic!
Every moment is so erratic!

Your bizarre concoctions never fail to amaze me!
Just a matter of letting the insight break free!
You suck that blandness out of life as if a bitter juice
You're just that crucial truce!

A park, a theatre or a party are magical
But, the wondrous human nature is equally fantastical!
The peculiarity of every soul
That throws a thousand question marks
in this curious mind!
As it sluggishly makes efforts to make them unwind.

Here is Power, there is Debility;
Here is Joy, there is Glee;
Here is Ignorance, there is Wisdom!
Diverse Colours, Countless Shades of You.
No wonder, You certainly make a brilliant composer!
As I get to perceive You even closer.

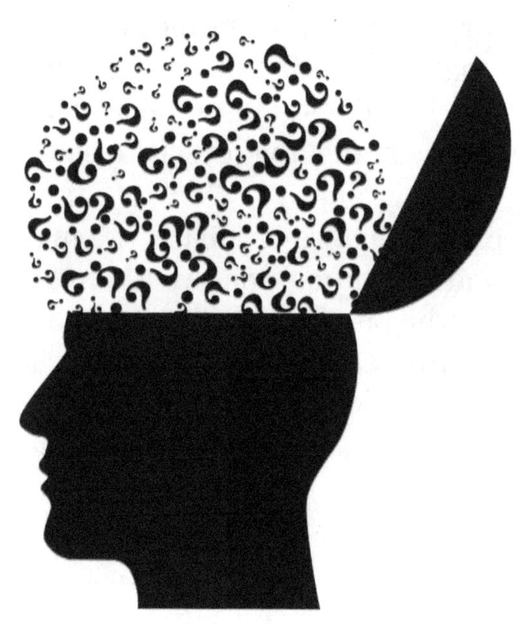

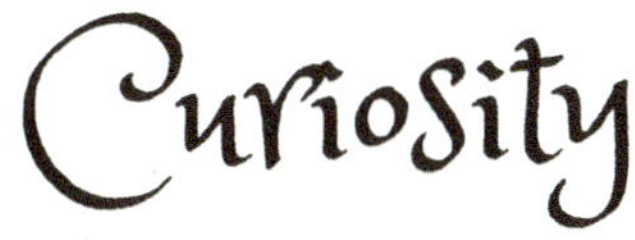

Curiosity

'Why, Who, Where, What, How' are Your best allies.
Who never fails to hassle me with their zealous sallies!

I confess You're the impetus for such sagacity.
But, today I ought to repine.
You presume I purport into an omniscient dabbler,
And also a proficient babbler!
Enough of those worthless tittle-tattles.
When it's followed by the muddling night rattles!

Are You a friend or a foe?
Though You let me grow, can I always be on my toes?

Off and on, senseless seems Your allies' notions.
Can You please redirect them to dive into the oceans?
An ocean of introspection, ocean of contemplation,
ocean of divine light!
Oh, this light would be so bright!
Can You envisage the glare of the celestial might?

I feel trailed; I quit.
As these queries are happily relinquished.
It's only then that the fire gets extinguished.
It's only then that the fire gets extinguished.

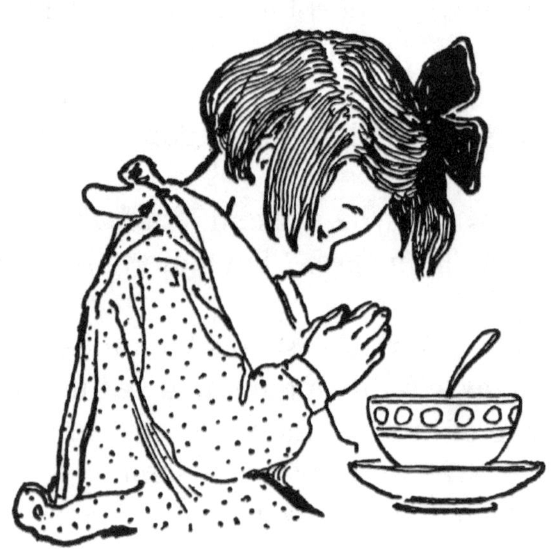

Gratitude

You ooze out the elixir of happiness!
That amazingly nullifies all the crappiness.

O my life, O my breaths, O my fate,
I love you, you're so great
There's nothing to equate
As this is my estate!

Addressing 'my' is so incredible.
All are priceless treasures. How impeccable!
The quirky cruces,
The arduous terrains.
How I was salvaged is ineffable!

What complaints, what resentments
when You always flow here
All evaporate to make the mind-sky clear!

You propel me to look around.
Disdain what I lack,
And all that is black.
Erase the nightmares,
Embrace the prayers.
Never mind, O my despair!
Never mind, O my despair!

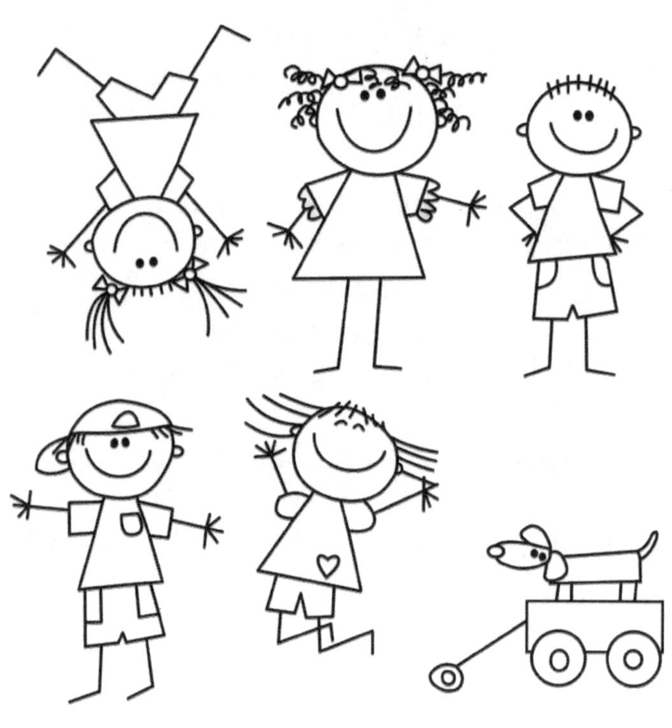

Happiness

O dear Happiness,
Every time I hold You tight,
You slip through my fingers.

Why are You so rude to me?
Every time I hold You tight,
You mercilessly leave me with a plea!

Such an Apathetic, are You?
Could You please spill on me like the drops of dew?

Where do You dwell?
Reveal Your abode
Is it somewhere concealed in those sweet memories?
Or in any victorious episode?
Do You reside in the canopy of Nature, the arms of a
Sojourn or the flavours of a cuisine?
Though radiant, I know it's just a rush of adrenaline!
You're there in a child's giggle, their naughty innocence.
But, I know You'll stay momentarily out of Your
insolence.

Alas, weary enough of my search for You,
Eventually, I got a glance at Your hue!
Oh, You mischievous playful flirt!
You were right there in the silence of my heart!
You were right there in the silence of my heart!

Rare emotions

They are rare.
But, be aware!
There may be a stare.
You might not care.
But, still there can be a flare!

Here is a brief about them.

1) Sonder: Everyone is a hero of their story
All can consider themselves as heroes
and heroines of their own life. This feeling suddenly
strikes me when I'm amidst a crowd where none of us
know each other. Still, all are part of the story of each
one! So strange yet true. The story where even if a
single face is missing from the reel, the story changes.

2) Zenosyne: Time keeps going faster
It's when I feel that time is running faster than my
thoughts.
It's when I want to be a kid and time takes me away to
adulthood. And this story continues lifelong.

3) Monachopsis: Being out of place
The odd one out is never welcomed. Individual brains,
individual choices, individual actions.

Still packed into the same frame by nature itself. Friction is ought to be produced when one of the surfaces match. So, this weird feeling of being out of place, being the odd one out. Still enjoying this scene as a game. But with a silent dream of landing into a land where similar hearts rejoice with me.

4) Lachesism: The desire to be struck by a disaster
The deep-seated wish that a disaster can only teach all of us. Teach us to care more about our Nature, care more about each other, care for the poor, etc.

5) Klexos: The Art of dwelling in the past
The past events are recalled as if this mind paints a picture where one event is correlated with another to form a bigger picture. The present picture of life seems so different without correlation with past events. So, as if there are two canvases of life. One that is perceived in the present. The other is the one that is formed after correlating all the past and present events.

6) Liberosis: The desire to care less about things
The more we are worried about things, the more they haunt us. So, it's this desire to let go, set free, leave everything to destiny and feel liberated.

7) Gnossienne: A moment of awareness that they too have a private life
I have known them for years. I have known about all the tiny secrets of their heart. Still, sometimes, it feels as if some hard-kept secrets dwell in their heart.

8) Jouska: Repeated hypothetical conversations of the mind
Though the conversation is over, this mind keeps on repeating the dialogues in the mind. 'I wish I had said that.', it whispers in my ears. Then slowly, it starts the whole conversation again in the mind. Lastly, it becomes silent only after it wins.

9) Enouement: The bittersweetness of arriving here in the future
An imagination where I can land in the future, literally. While some of the events appear sweet as so many unanswered questions finally get an answer. But at the same time, it can be a bitter feeling as I can see the blunders I've made these years. And the perceptions break as pieces of glass!

10) Kuebiko: Exhausted by acts of senseless violence
A scene of violent acts, riots flashes in front of me. Why, what, where, how pops up immediately. The questions are without answers. Still, I am bound to witness those acts of violence. Though I have the urge to help the people, it seems impossible.

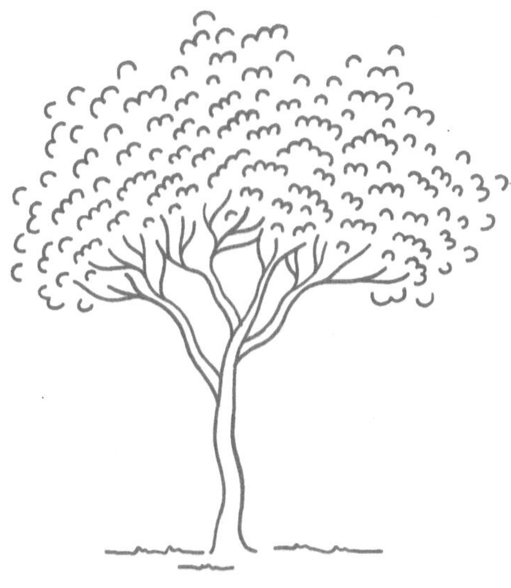

Sonder

Everyone has a story

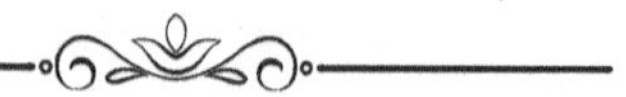

I was blithesome taking a walk around the hills.
A pleasant day with a rejuvenating picnic and some
chilling thrills!
Suddenly, You poked me.
And I vanished into Your profound colours.
I could see a grand screenplay.
I was the supreme patron all set to enter the fray!
Thousands of minions around.
Each of them boast of being crowned!

Family and friends, seniors and juniors, friends and
foes,
All together filled those vivid colours to this beautiful
canvas.
One colour departs for an exile,
And the canvas is vile!
Please excuse me for being selfish!
As I ought to have all of them.
More and more colours,
More and more folks.
With every breath that I take in.
With every step that I move in.

Suddenly, I could see my look alike!
Nature's stunning plans, I guessed.
Instantly, visuals of me in her shoe flashes.
Oh, again I'm the veteran
The associates are perfectly in their roles.
The passerby I stumbled upon was me!
'Oh, I'm sorry', I said and moved on.
That was all the interplay between us.
That was all the interplay between us.

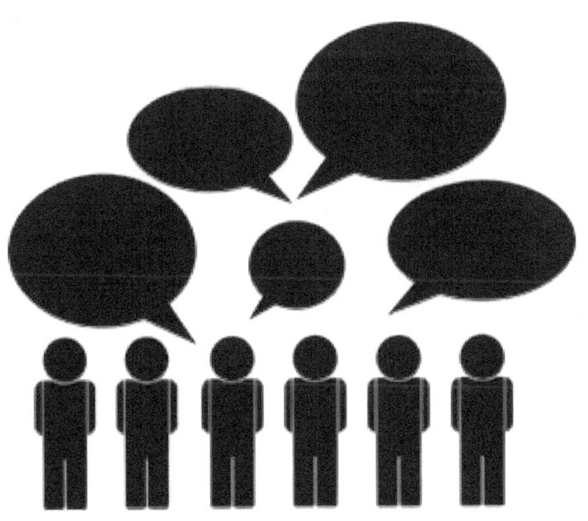

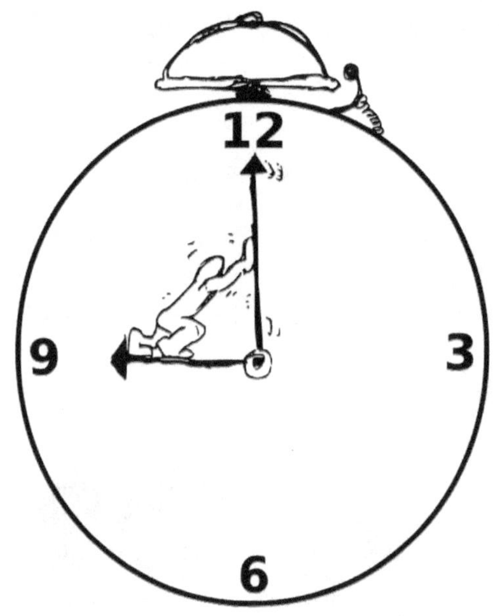

Gossiping with my emotions

Zenosyne

Time keeps going faster

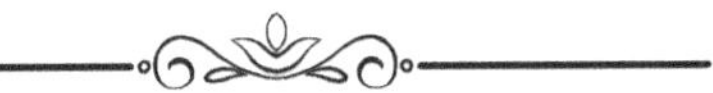

A flying time gently whispers.
'Come fly with me.
Sorry to announce.
But You ought to renounce.
Do You have any choice?
It was all of such rejoice.'

The child wished to play.
But was abducted by the flying jalopy.
And dumped into the adolescent canopy.
Just as the juvenile colours sprinkled all over,
It was time for a crossover!

Let me switch it off so that it sets off a standstill.
But, such a sagacious Creator that my dial control is
nil!
With hands tied up and a mourning heart,
Every scene is witnessed.
With every moment that passes,
With every bond with their quirky splashes,
With every joy and sorrow embraced,
I wish You could be replaced.
I wish You were a fantasy.
But You're a reality.
I'm coerced to embrace.
I'm coerced to embrace.

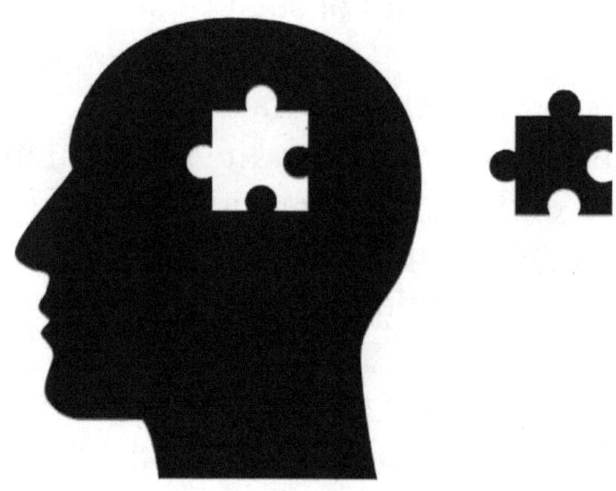

Monachopsis

Being out of place

Dead amongst the living.
Live amongst the dead.
Fire amongst ice cubes.
Chilling ice amongst burning fumes.

Whom to blame?
That we are in the same frame!
Is it fair to disclaim?
Why exclaim?
Such a wonderful game!

One moment I'm here. The other I'm with You.
How long do I Camouflage?
Why this intention to sabotage!
Sabotage this alien sphere.
Before I disappear!
Only to reappear.

Reappear in a pally vista.
Relishing a grand fiesta!
Amidst those palsy-walsy faces.
Where I breathe free rein.
Where I love to mellow out again and again.
Where my fluid steps are on the move.
As if they love to behove.
In this intimate, cosy home.
In this intimate, cosy home.

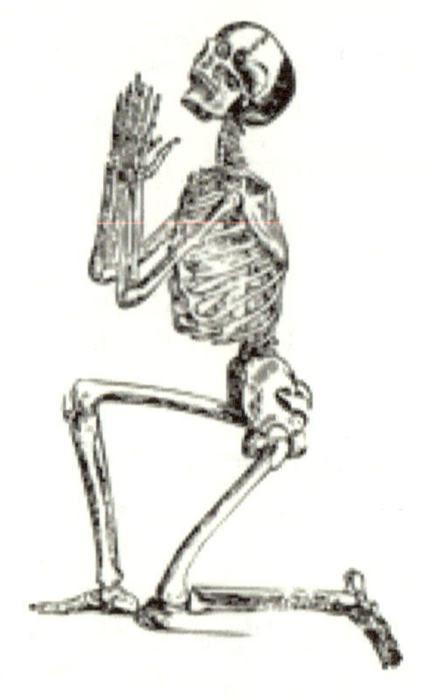

Lachesism

The desire to be struck by a disaster

'As you sow, so shall you reap.'
A dictum we ought to prove.

When we are least bothered by the deteriorating Gaia.
When we are nonchalant at the sight of the penniless.
When we abort our conscience!

Oh, Your love for a quiz!
Are You a justice wiz?

You bombard those hundreds of questions.
You're the question. You're the answer.
An answer that isn't a sweet dish.
But, an answer for which I unexpectedly wish!

A wish for a disaster!
With tons of those blasters!

A wish for a turbulent storm that washes away all the
sins.
Gosh, a moment of rejoicing when truth wins!

A wish for a tutor.
Who's also a prosecutor.

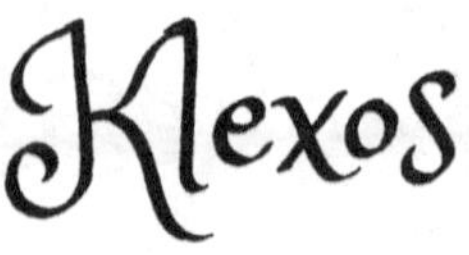

Klexos

The Art of dwelling in the past

Two canvases of this life.
One unfolds this moment. The other is a masterpiece!
Eidetic images flow effortlessly on the screen!
You're behind that facial sheen!

One picture of this moment.
Always baffling.
The other of the bygone moments.
Always enlightening!

The Past Canvas.
Painted to narrate a story.
A story, a journey.
A journey from concealment to revelation.
A journey from mystification to clarification.
A journey from yesterday to today.
The destination is where the canvases converge.
And start a new journey.
From today to tomorrow.
That again paints a canvas.
From yesterday to today.

What do I call this weird feeling?
It's neither regret nor nostalgia.
It's You, the ceaseless, indefatigable painter!
How amazing are your colours?
That is never exhausted.
That is never repeated.

There's Vibrance!
There's Elegance!
Such a Remembrance,
With absolute Transparency
With absolute Transparency.

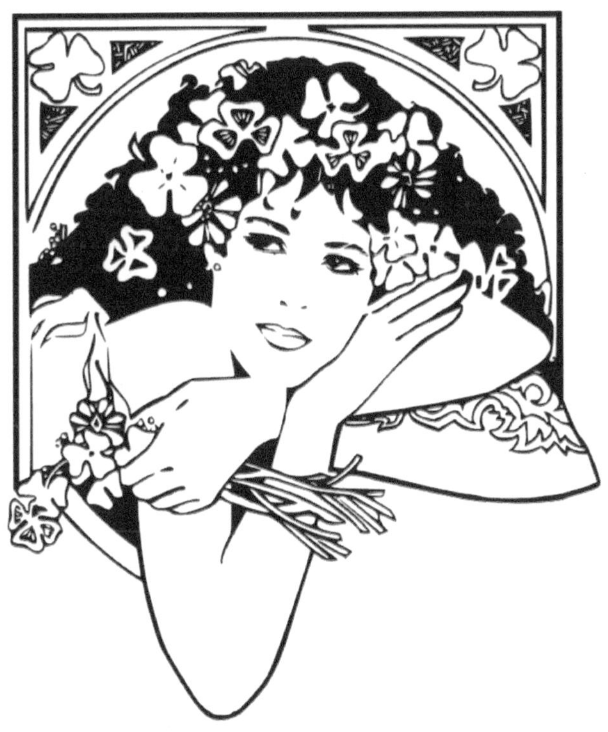

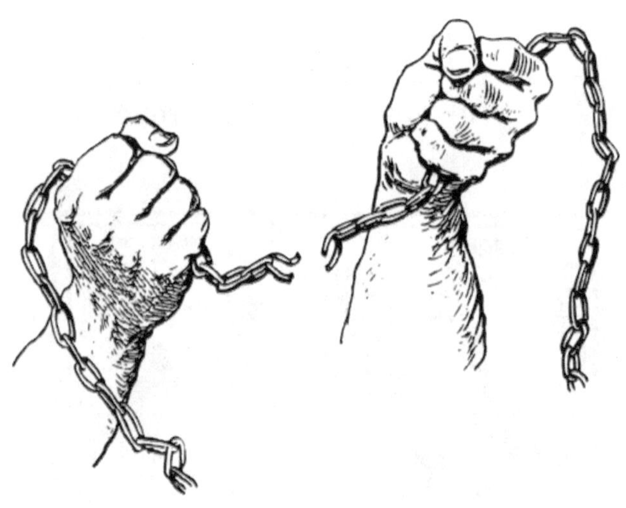

Gossiping with my emotions

Liberosis

The desire to care less about things

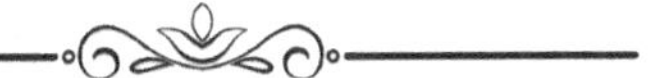

Oh, this bosom yearning for sovereignty!
The shackles come alive to tighten with great velocity!
Surely, it's their aristocracy!
Shackles of desires.
Shackles of relationships.
Shackles of responsibilities.
Shackles of fear.
Libertas!
Dimittas!
Gliding in the air.
With all the hefty cargo shed off with that tear.

Now, I see those pally tides and ebbs.
Now, I see those pally insecurities.
Now, I see those pally puzzles.
Drifting lightly in that soft breeze.
Unfazed.
Unstirred.
Tranquillized!
'Oh, Life! You're unrestrained now.
Ready to be challenged?
Hope all the nasty will be scavenged.'

Gnossienne

**A moment of awareness
that they too have a private life**

The mansion of his heart.
Thousands of memories. Thousands of rooms.
I've danced in all except for one.

My corridors, my lounge.
Where I love to linger as I've been crowned!
My stretch where the lord of the manor never frowned.

One knock at the doors and here's a grand escort!
Affirmations, genuine concerns, always ready to exhort!
But why is that door always with a bolt?
Is it a reservoir of an insult or flashpoint of a revolt?

Imaginations can only unfurl into these eyes.
Hope to burst open that door, hear those cries!
When You poke me at that ecstatic moment.
And choke the jovial bestowment!
As I've danced in all, except for one.
As I've danced in all, except for one.

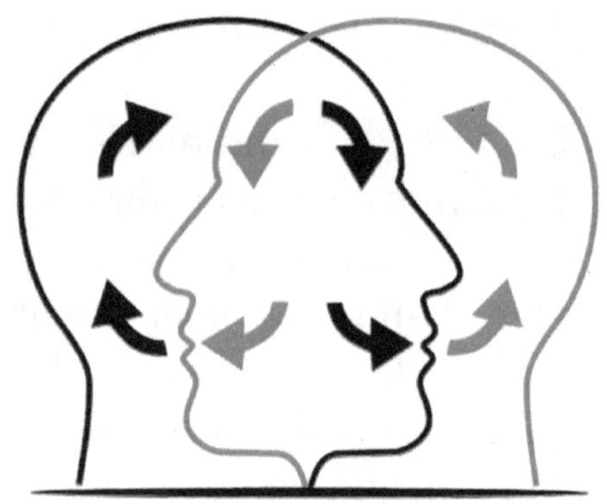

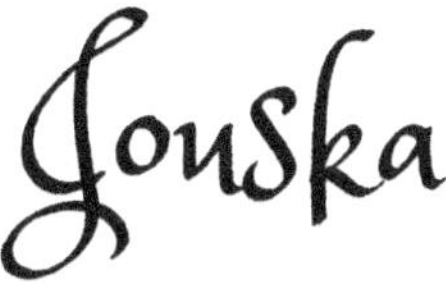

Repeated hypothetical conversations of the mind

You're such a colossal chatterer!
A sly fox, a flatterer!

The dialogues have been staged.
Isn't it too late to be enraged!
Is there an exigency for the offenders to be savaged?

A prosecutor jumping into the court of the mind.
The sense of time and sentience left behind.
And here goes the screenplay!

An eloquent script.
What a fiery afflict!
A speechless convict!
Alas, the resolved conflict.
A victor is here, albeit illusory!

You were the judge, restless to announce the
percipience
Surely, it's time for resilience.
Gosh, now the ears are experiencing silence.
Gosh, now the ears are experiencing silence.

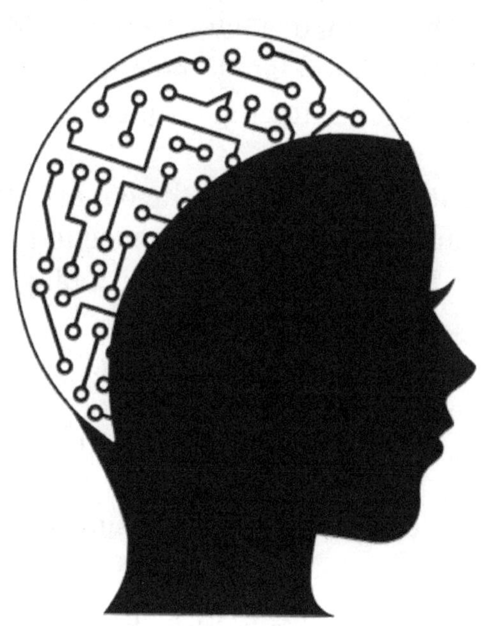

Gossiping with my emotions

82

Enouement

The bittersweetness of arriving here in the future

The wheel of time rolls.
And it rolls faster.
And it rolls the fastest.
The skyjack with the zephyr.

Voila! I'm in the future.
Incredulity! Bewilderment! Consternation!
Solved equations.
Answered questions.
Mystifying answers.
Or a new set of questions?
Abandoned for You to answer!

A highly uncontested decision was a blunder!
A friend emerges as a foe. What a wonder!
Anticipations, postulations, presuppositions.
'Such Irrationals' is Your declaration!

All bets are off.
A trusted dumbling pop out as a genius.
A trusted genius warrants as a dumbling.
Fiction and reality are in concord.
What is fiction?
What is reality?
You are the silent omniscient novelist.

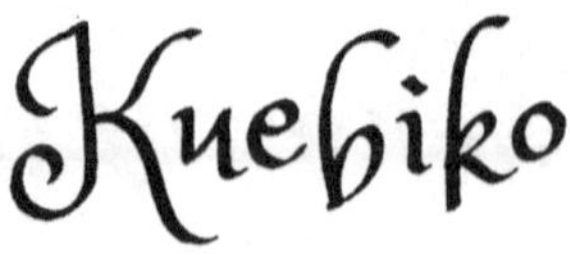

Kuebiko

Exhaustion by acts of senseless violence

The ferocious fights, the mindless squabbles.
Alack, this head is blasé about those wobbles!

A utopian world.
With an eternal progression.
All with perfection.
Suddenly it is an illusion!
Smashed by such aggression.
A giant brain
And a miniature heart!
Where bodies are torn apart!

A cluttered heart
Craves a cleanse
The untold intent
Are suddenly ever ready to portend.

The intent to wipe
And resolve this nasty hype.
Alas, the intent lacks guts.
To reveal the silliness to the mutts!

So I'm here as a statue
Whether a scorching heat or dew.
Powerless to ignite a revolution
Powerless to move either!
How to spin the head when the pals are dying!
How to look around either!

Let me be there deaf, blind and mute
Let me just be there deaf, blind and mute.

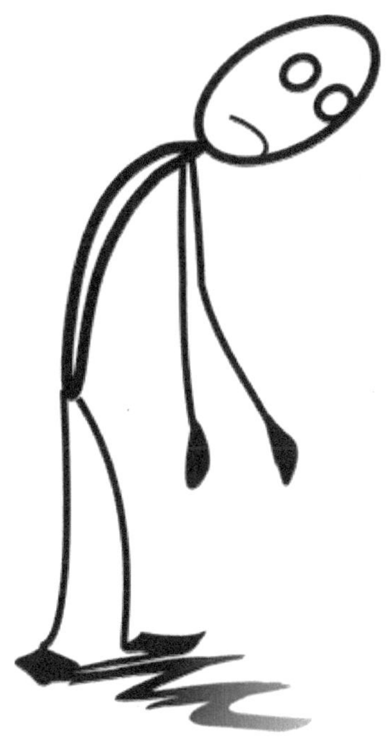

Self-test for Emotional Quotient

1) a} Are you unable to consciously change your mood whenever you want and

   b} Are you unable to sense other people's moods?
   - Yes
   - No

2) Do you feel other people (not your family members) are difficult to understand and you find them very different from your own emotional circle?
   - Yes
   - No
   - Can't Say

3) Do you feel angry when someone finds nooks in your work?
- Yes
- No
- Can't say
- Sometimes

4) Do you feel irritated to wait for someone for a while?
- Yes
- No
- Can't say
- Sometimes

5) Do you feel discomfort in contacting some of the past relations?

- Yes
- No
- May be

[If your answer is Yes in most of the questions, then it's time for you to upgrade your EQ (Emotional Quotient) level.
If your answer is No in most of the questions, your EQ (Emotional Quotient) level is bang on or high.
If your answer is Can't say, Sometimes or May be in most of the questions, you need to have an introspection about your own emotions]

6) How would you react in the following situation?

Your senior, boss or elder person has scolded you badly. And you've got an important event to attend where the same person who scolded you is also going to be present. And you have to deliver a speech and attend some guests. Now what would you most likely do?

A) It would be very easy for you to be cheerful in the event.

B) You'll take 1-2 hours to become normal and attend the event.

C) You may have an argument with someone in the event.

D) You'll ignore the person who scolded you in the party

[If your answer is A) Your EQ level is high
If your answer is B) Your EQ level is pretty good enough though you can improve it.
If your answer is C) Your EQ level is low and you need to urgently work on it.
If your answer is D) Your EQ level is on an average level and there's scope for improvement.

7) What would you do in the following situation?
Someone you loved so much has just betrayed you. You
had put your life at stake for that one person. And today
he or she is gone from your life.
There are no options for this question. Take a pen and
paper and start writing the answer. I'm sure you'll get
the answer. An answer that doesn't make others cry as
you've cried for that loss. An answer for the betterment
of you and your family. An answer that calls for a shoot
in your EQ (Emotional Quotient).

{Important Declaration:

This questionnaire can be used as a tool for a self-test
to assess your emotional intelligence or emotional
quotient when put in difficult situations.
This intelligence gives you the power to pro-actively
sense the inner turmoil, analyze it and uproot it out.
This is not only important in today's hectic lifestyle but
also necessary to save all those priceless relationships
that we often take it for granted.
This intelligence acts like a mental shield to protect you
from all the inner turmoil that becomes the basis for all
those insensible words and actions that we have regret
for.
So, take your first step to improve your EQ. Take your
first step to question your inner being. Be honest. Be
yourself.}

<u>Notes for self</u>

- ....
- ....
- ....
- ....
- ....
- ....

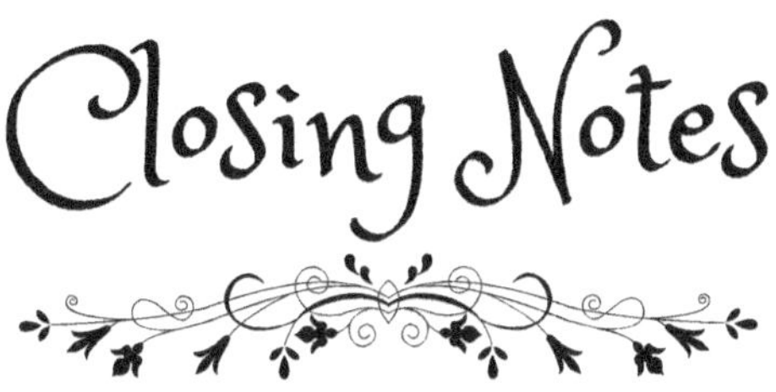

Closing Notes

Congratulations readers! You have succeeded to enhance your EQ (Emotional Quotient).

Here, I would like to let you know a fact that any burst of emotion (or the biological chemicals) in the body takes just 4-7 seconds to spread in the whole body. That means you just have 4-7 seconds to be aware of what emotion you're going through and curb them. So, if you know your emotions better it would be easier for you to curb them because 4-7 seconds of your life can sometimes cost you an important relationship.

Here, I would also like to convey my earnest thanks to you. I've written how I have felt about any particular emotion. You may have your own experience. Thanks for connecting so well to my experiences.

A humble request to make an easy-to-execute plan. Take a pen and paper at the end of the day. Write down your feelings about any particular person, thing, place or event that you've experienced during the day. Break free all the boundaries when you write as you're writing for yourself. It's only then that you can truly know about your heart picture.

"Everything is created twice, first in the mind and then in reality." - Robin Sharma

"If you don't mind, it doesn't matter." - Jack Benny
In other words, what you think decides how you feel. And that ultimately becomes your reality.
Here's a YouTube channel initiated by me that very humbly tries to improve mental health through spirituality where 'happier you, happier life' is the motto. Just have a look through the link given below.

https://youtube.com/c/spiritualdose4u

Altenatively, you could visit the below social medial platforms as well.

Quora   https://healthynspiritualindia.quora.com/

facebook https://www.facebook.com/Healthynspiritual

Instagram health_and_spiritual_india